# BEST WAYS TO ~~ADHD~~ ADHD IN TEENS AND YOUNG ADULTS

## Empowering Young Minds; Effective Approaches for Successful Parenting in ADHD Teens and Young Adults

### *(Inspirational stories included)*

**Dr. Richard J. Kay**

# Copyright

# Table of contents

# Chapter 1

# Introduction

## Understanding ADHD in Children and Adolescents

ADHD is a complex neurodevelopmental condition that affects millions of teens and young adults worldwide. But what exactly is it?

## What Exactly Is ADHD?

Attention Deficit Hyperactivity illness (ADHD) is a neurodevelopmental illness that affects a person's ability to focus, control impulses, and regulate their attention and energy levels. It is more than just being hyper or having a short attention span; it is a multidimensional condition that can present itself in a variety of ways.

Understanding the complexities of ADHD is critical. It is not a one-size-fits-all illness, with symptoms varying from individual to person. Some people battle primarily with inattention, while others struggle with hyperactivity and impulsivity. It's more than just a "short attention span"; it's a complicated interplay of cognitive and behavioral issues.

## ADHD prevalence among adolescents

You are not by yourself. ADHD is one of the most frequently diagnosed mental health problems among adolescents. It is estimated that 8-10% of children and adolescents suffer from ADHD. That equates to one or two students in each course! Understanding the prevalence of ADHD is important because it reminds us that it is not an isolated problem; it is a shared experience for many people, and there is a wealth of collective knowledge and support to draw on.

## ADHD's Biological Basis

What factors contribute to ADHD? For years, scholars have been intrigued by this question. While we don't know everything, we do know that ADHD has a biological basis. Neuroimaging studies have revealed abnormalities in brain structure and function in ADHD patients. Dopamine and norepinephrine, in particular, play an important role in ADHD, influencing attention, motivation, and impulse control.

Understanding the biological basis of ADHD is similar to having a road map for the condition. It explains why some treatments work, why medicine can be a successful treatment, and why ADHD does not simply go away with age.

## ADHD Myths & Misconceptions

Before we get into the meat of ADHD management in teens and young adults, it's critical to dispel some prevalent myths and misconceptions. These myths can lead to stigma and misunderstandings about ADHD, making it difficult for individuals to receive the necessary assistance and understanding.

One common misconception is that ADHD is caused by inadequate parenting or a lack of discipline. Nothing could be further from the truth. ADHD is a neurological condition that parents cannot "cure" through better discipline. It's also not a condition that children outgrow; it frequently persists into adulthood.

Another myth is that medication is a "quick fix" or that taking medication means giving up on non-pharmacological interventions. In actuality, medication can be a vital tool in an ADHD management plan, but it's just one piece of the puzzle. Non-medical strategies, such counseling, lifestyle adjustments, and educational support, are equally important and are typically used in conjunction with medicine.

As we progress through this book, we'll continue to debunk myths and replace them with facts, laying the groundwork for you to navigate the world of ADHD more effectively.

## The Importance of Proper ADHD Management

Understanding ADHD is the first step, but it is only the starting point. The importance of effective ADHD management is at the heart of our discussion.

ADHD, like any other medical condition, demands a careful and proactive approach to guarantee individuals may thrive despite its limitations. The impact of ADHD extends beyond academic or professional performance; it impacts personal relationships, self-esteem, and overall well-being. Effective ADHD management can make a lot of difference in these areas.

ADHD doesn't have to be a hindrance to achievement; it may be a source of strength. Many very successful people, ranging from entrepreneurs and artists to athletes and academics, have used the unique characteristics of ADHD to achieve greatness. This promise can be realized with effective management.

## Overview of the Book

So, what are your expectations for this book? "How to Handle ADHD in teens and Young Adults" is designed to be your partner on this path. It's not a one-size-fits-all solution but a toolkit filled with ideas, insights, and tales to assist you or your loved one manage life with ADHD.

In the chapters that follow, we will delve into the diagnosis and identification of ADHD, explore the role of medication and other therapies, discuss academic performance, and focus on establishing key life skills. We'll dive into themes like healthy living, stress management, and goal planning, arming you with the tools needed to excel in all parts of life.

This book is an inspiration as well as a source of information. Throughout the chapters, you'll come across real-life examples of people who have not only managed with ADHD, but have transformed it into a strength. You'll find practical information, strategies, and techniques for overcoming typical ADHD issues.

We strive to deliver up-to-date information by integrating scientific insights with practical advice. While ADHD is a lifelong diagnosis, it is one that can be efficiently managed, and this book will help you get there.

So let us begin this trip together. There's something here for everyone, whether you're an adolescent, young adult, parent, teacher, or friend. We can unlock the potential that exists within every individual living with ADHD with a dash of understanding, a pinch of patience, and a sprinkle of dedication. Let us embark on the journey of thriving with ADHD rather than despite it, and flip the page to a brighter future.

## Inspirational Story

*Welcome to the book "How to Handle ADHD in Teens and Young Adults. " In the following pages, we will go on a journey to better understand Attention Deficit Hyperactivity Disorder (ADHD) in teenagers and young adults. ADHD is a complicated, diverse disorder that can present difficulties, but it can also be a source of unique abilities and talents. As we progress through this book, we will investigate the complexities of ADHD and provide you with the information and tools to not just manage it well, but to thrive with it.*

## ADHD in Adolescents and Young Adults:

*Let me begin by introducing you to Sarah, a 17-year-old high school student who has been diagnosed with ADHD from childhood. Sarah's life is a frenzy of homework, extracurricular activities, and attempting to fit in with her classmates. Her teachers frequently found her inattentive, forgetful, and occasionally unruly at school, which led to some early misunderstandings. Despite her apparent difficulties, Sarah is a remarkably creative, quick-witted, and sensitive individual. She hasn't, however, fully realized the potential of her special powers.*

*ADHD is a lived experience, not just a clinical diagnosis. As we put ourselves in Sarah's shoes, we'll look at the problems she experiences on a daily basis. The emotional rollercoaster, the trouble* concentration, and the nagging sense of inadequacy are all part of the ADHD landscape. But we'll also uncover Sarah's limitless energy, vivid creativity, and capacity to think beyond the box.

Sarah's tale is not unusual. Millions of teenagers and young adults suffer from ADHD, and each has their own experience. We can begin to unlock the potential of ADHD by knowing these distinct experiences.

### The Importance of Proper ADHD Management:

Let's take a step back and look at the larger picture. ADHD is not a one-size-fits-all condition, and its impact on individuals varies greatly. When we consider how ADHD impacts not only Sarah but also her family, teachers, and friends, the need for proper ADHD management becomes clear. It's not just about Sarah; it's about providing a nurturing environment for her.

*Effective ADHD management begins with understanding that ADHD is not a restriction, but rather a different way of experiencing the world. It is about devising strategies that will assist Sarah in staying on top of her assignments, completing her chores, and navigating her social interactions. More importantly, it is about developing self-esteem, resilience, and self-advocacy skills that will serve her for the rest of her life.*

## Summary of the book:

In the following chapters, we will delve into ADHD in teenagers and young adults, combining cutting-edge scientific research with practical, real-world advice. We'll look at how to diagnose ADHD, build a support network, and decide on the best treatment approach, whether medication or alternative methods are used. We'll delve into the critical domains of academic success and life skills, assisting individuals like Sarah in better managing their daily routines. We'll also discuss the importance of living a healthy lifestyle, which includes good eating, exercise, and stress management.

We'll help Sarah and others develop and achieve significant goals, whether in school, at work, or in their personal lives. Another key issue we will discuss is the transition to adulthood, which will ensure that teenagers with ADHD are well-prepared for independence.

Throughout this book, we'll tell the tales of people like Sarah who have learned to use their ADHD abilities to achieve in life. We hope that these remarkable stories will inspire and empower our readers.

Our goal is to deliver an entertaining and dynamic experience that encourages readers to investigate, contemplate, and build tactics adapted to their individual circumstances. Whether you're a teen with ADHD, a parent, an educator, or a healthcare professional, this book is a wonderful resource for making life with ADHD not only manageable but also enjoyable.

So, let us go on this trip together, learning how to thrive with ADHD as we read Best Ways to Handle ADHD in Teens and Young Adults"

# Chapter 2

# Recognising ADHD

In the previous chapter, we looked into the fundamentals of ADHD, knowing its definition, prevalence, and the biological underpinnings of this complicated neurodevelopmental illness. Now, let's go even deeper into the world of ADHD by focusing on recognition—recognising ADHD in teens and young adults.

## Common Symptoms and Behaviour

ADHD is commonly classified as a "hidden" condition, and for good reason. Its symptoms can be modest, easily dismissed, or attributed to other circumstances. But once we know what to look for, ADHD becomes significantly less elusive. Let's study the common signs and behaviors connected with ADHD, which will help in its recognition.

## The Core Symptoms of ADHD

ADHD can be broken down into three basic symptom groups, and individuals with ADHD may experience a combination of these:

a. **Inattentiveness**: A hallmark of ADHD, inattentiveness, entails problems sustaining attention, forgetfulness, frequent casual mistakes, and trouble organizing tasks. These actions typically lead to missing details, a tendency to be easily distracted, and challenges in following through with activities.

b. **Hyperactivity**: Hyperactivity is characterized by restlessness and the inability to sit motionless for an extended period of time. It can cause fidgeting, tapping, or continual movement, making it difficult to focus or perform calm, immobile jobs.

c. **Impulsivity**: Impulsivity is defined as the inclination to act without considering the consequences. People with ADHD may interrupt others, have difficulty waiting their turn, or speak and act quickly, which can lead to misunderstandings and rash actions.

## The Varying Expressions of ADHD

It is critical to recognise that ADHD is not a one-size-fits-all condition. Individuals with ADHD have personalities and behavior that differ from those who do not have ADHD. ADHD presents differently in each person, resulting in diverse manifestations of the disorder. This variety can make it difficult to identify ADHD, but it also emphasizes the significance of tailored screening and care.

## Hidden Struggles

People with ADHD may develop coping techniques or compensate for their difficulties in some instances. This can obscure their symptoms, making them even more difficult to identify. A teen with ADHD, for example, may be exceptionally bright yet struggle in school due to difficulty with focus or organization. A young adult with ADHD may excel at work while struggling with inward restlessness.

Understanding these hidden difficulties and the various manifestations of ADHD is the first step towards recognising it. Here are some practical indicators and behavior to look out for in teens and young adults to help you better detect ADHD:

# Practical Signs to Watch For

- **Academic concerns**: Common homework concerns such as forgetfulness, disorganization, and trouble completing assignments. There is frequently a considerable disparity between an individual's potential and their actual performance.

- **Inconsistent Performance**: A person with ADHD may succeed in areas of great interest while struggling in others. For both the individual and those around them, inconsistency can be bewildering.

- **Time Management Struggles:** Difficulties estimating and managing time can lead to chronic lateness, missed appointments, and frantic, last-minute work.

- **Impulsivity**: is characterized by frequent outbursts in conversations, acting without thinking, and difficulties waiting one's turn in social activities.

- **Inadequate Organization:** chronic disorganization, clutter, and difficulties keeping a tidy workstation or personal living area.

- **Mood Swings**: Individuals with ADHD may experience more dramatic emotional shifts. Irritability, frustration, and short tempers are typical.

- **Procrastination**: A procrastination pattern can be seen in daily duties, homework assignments, and employment responsibilities.

- **Inconsistent Focus:** Difficulty remaining engaged in tasks, particularly those that are repetitious or demand sustained concentration.

- **Frequent Forgetfulness**: lapses in memory that lead to missed appointments, forgotten obligations, and misplaced items

- **Restlessness**: Hyperactivity can be characterized by a difficulty to sit still, frequent fidgeting, or excessive movement.

- **Difficulty Listening**: The inability to pay attention during conversations, lectures, or meetings, especially when the information is critical.

## Diagnosis and Assessment

Recognising the signs and habits linked with ADHD is a vital first step, but it is also critical to understand that a formal diagnosis is required. A professional diagnosis confirms the presence of ADHD and helps select the best therapy and support.

## The Diagnosis Procedure

Several critical steps are usually involved in the diagnostic process:

a. **Clinical Assessment**: A full clinical assessment will be performed by a healthcare provider, most likely a psychiatrist, pediatrician, or neurologist. They will gather information from parents, teachers, and other sources regarding the individual's medical history, development, and behavior.

b. **ADHD Rating Scales**: Standardized ADHD rating scales are frequently used to assess the presence and severity of symptoms. These questionnaires are completed by parents, teachers, or the individual.

c. **Rule-Out Process:** The healthcare professional will also look for other disorders that may be mistaken for or co-occur with ADHD, such as anxiety, depression, or learning difficulties. It's critical to rule out any other possible reasons for the symptoms you're experiencing.

d. **Observation**: During the evaluation, the healthcare professional may examine the individual's behaviors to assess their attention, impulse control, and hyperactivity.

e. **Criteria Assessment**: The diagnosis of ADHD is based on certain criteria outlined in the American Psychiatric Association's Diagnostic and Statistical Manual of Mental Disorders (DSM-5). To be diagnosed with ADHD, a person must match the criteria described in this document.

f. **Feedback and Discussion**: The healthcare provider will go over the assessment results with the individual and their family. They will explain whether an ADHD diagnosis is appropriate and what measures to take next.

# The Importance of Early Detection

For various reasons, early detection and diagnosis of ADHD are critical. First and foremost, a proper diagnosis allows individuals and their families to gain access to the support and resources they require to effectively manage ADHD.

Many of the difficulties associated with ADHD can be avoided or reduced with early intervention, whether in school, at work, or in personal relationships. Early understanding of the disease can also assist parents and carers in tailoring their approach to provide the greatest support for their kid.

Furthermore, early detection helps lessen the chance of secondary disorders, such as low self-esteem, anxiety, and depression, which frequently accompany untreated ADHD. Individuals can begin to develop the skills and techniques needed to thrive by addressing ADHD as soon as possible.

Remember that identifying ADHD is only the first step. A proper diagnosis and extensive assessment are required for the development of a customized management plan that allows people with ADHD to attain their full potential.

We've now looked at the most prevalent symptoms and behavior related to ADHD, as well as the diagnostic process. In the next chapters, we'll look at techniques and therapies for effectively managing ADHD in teens and young adults, ensuring they not only cope but thrive despite the disease.

To demonstrate the concepts from Chapter 2, let us enter the life of Sarah, a 16-year-old high school student.

## Inspirational Story

*Sarah is a vibrant and inventive young woman who has always been full of life. Her parents referred to her as a "free spirit" since she demonstrated remarkable creativity, an insatiable curiosity about the world, and unlimited energy from an early age. However, as she approached adolescence, her parents began to detect some troubling patterns.*

### Common Signs and Symptoms

*Sarah's parents saw that while she excelled in topics she was interested in, such as art and literature, she struggled to focus and complete her homework in others. Her room was a frenzy of creativity, but it was* also chaotic. Homework projects were frequently strewn about and forgotten, buried beneath a mound of art supplies.

She frequently interrupted talks at home and at school, blurting out her opinions on the spur of the moment. Her impulsiveness caused unpleasant occasions in social contexts. Despite her bright mind and amazing potential, her academic performance was uneven, causing both her and her parents to be frustrated.

## Diagnosis and Evaluation

Sarah's parents decided to seek professional help after reading about ADHD and seeing some of the signs in her. They arranged an appointment with a neurodevelopmental problem specialist child psychologist. The psychologist did a thorough evaluation that included interviews with Sarah, her parents, and her teachers.

*Sarah's parents completed ADHD rating measures, and her teachers were interviewed about her behavior in class. During the assessment, the psychologist also watched Sarah's behaviors. Sarah found it difficult to sit still and frequently fidgeted in her chair. During the evaluation, she struggled to focus on the activities at hand and demonstrated impulsive behaviors.*

*The assessment assisted the psychologist in ruling out other potential illnesses and indicated that Sarah fitted the DSM-5 criteria for an ADHD diagnosis.*

## Early Detection and Assistance

*Sarah and her parents had a range of feelings following the diagnosis, including relief, affirmation, and some worry. They immediately realized, however, the necessity of early detection and intervention.*

*Sarah's parents were able to work closely with the school to adopt solutions to meet her academic requirements after receiving a confirmed ADHD diagnosis. Among these strategies was a 504 Plan, which provided accommodations such as extra time on examinations and a quiet workstation. Sarah also started working with a qualified tutor who assisted her with organization and time management.*

*Sarah and her parents investigated non-medical methods, such as cognitive-behavioral therapy, with the support of her psychologist to help her manage impulsivity and improve her organizational abilities. Sarah progressively learned how to harness her creativity and energy while managing her symptoms as a result of these interventions, which helped her recognise her unique strengths and limitations.*

*Recognising Sarah's ADHD was only the beginning of her journey. Despite her ADHD, she began to thrive with early intervention and specialized assistance. Sarah's creative hobbies continued to flourish as the years passed, and her academic skills progressively improved. She accepted her ADHD as part of what made her distinctive and learned to capitalize on its strengths.*

*Sarah's experience emphasizes the need of diagnosing ADHD symptoms, receiving an official diagnosis, and seeking the required assistance and interventions to assist teens and young people like her in reaching their full potential. ADHD is not a barrier to achievement; in fact, it may be a source of strength and resilience when used correctly.*

# Chapter 3

# Treatment Options

In Chapter 2, we discussed how to recognise ADHD, its prevalent symptoms, and the significance of receiving an official diagnosis. Now we'll look at ADHD treatment options for teenagers and young adults. Effective management is essential for thriving with ADHD, and a variety of strategies are available to assist individuals in harnessing their unique strengths while addressing their challenges.

## Medication Administration

Medication is one of the most well-known and well-researched therapy choices for ADHD. But what exactly is medication management, and how does it function?

# How to Understand ADHD Medications

ADHD medications are classified into two types: stimulants and non-stimulants. While the term "stimulant" may seem counterintuitive, these medications are effective in improving focus and impulse control in ADHD patients.

The most commonly prescribed medications are stimulants such as methylphenidate (e.g., Ritalin) and amphetamine-based drugs (e.g., Adderall). They function by raising the brain's concentrations of certain neurotransmitters, such dopamine and norepinephrine. These neurotransmitters are essential for attention, motivation, and impulse control.

Non-stimulant medications, such as atomoxetine (Strattera) and guanfacine (Intuniv), work differently than stimulant medications and should be considered when stimulant medications are ineffective or have undesirable side effects.

## Medication's Effectiveness

ADHD medications are not a cure for the condition, but they can be an effective tool in managing it. Medication has been shown in studies to improve focus, attention, and impulse control in people with ADHD. When the proper drug and dosage are found, many people notice improvements in their academic or professional performance, personal relationships, and overall quality of life.

It is crucial to note that pharmaceutical effectiveness varies from person to person. What suits one individual may probably not suit another. Finding the proper drug and dosage may necessitate some patience and close coordination with a healthcare specialist.

## Potential Side Effects and Considerations

Like other treatments, ADHD meds come with possible adverse effects. Common adverse effects of stimulant drugs can include increased heart rate, decreased appetite, and difficulties sleeping. Non-stimulant drugs may have distinct adverse effects, such as sleepiness and changes in blood pressure.

It's crucial to work closely with a healthcare provider to monitor and manage any adverse effects. They can change the medicine kind, dose, or timing to find the greatest balance between symptom control and side effect minimisation.

## Behavioral Therapies

In addition to medication management, behavioral therapies play a significant role in helping individuals with ADHD develop skills to cope with their symptoms. These therapies are often used in conjunction with medicine to provide a comprehensive approach to treatment.

## Cognitive-Behavioral Therapy (CBT)

Cognitive-behavioral therapy is a well-established strategy that helps individuals with ADHD notice and overcome harmful thought patterns and behaviors. It is extremely helpful for controlling impulsive behavior, enhancing organization and time management, and decreasing emotional reactivity.

Individuals learn to recognise triggers for impulsive behaviors and acquire ways to pause and make more deliberate decisions during CBT sessions. They also concentrate on defining and accomplishing short- and long-term objectives, which can be very beneficial for teenagers and young adults.

## Parent Training

Parent training is an excellent resource for children and adolescents with ADHD. These programmes give parents techniques and tools to help them properly manage their child's ADHD symptoms. Setting clear and consistent goals, providing positive reinforcement, and building an organized and supportive home environment are all common components of parent training.

## Social Skills Training

Inattention and impulsivity might impair a person's ability to handle social situations. Individuals who receive social skills training improve their interpersonal abilities, which are required to form and maintain relationships. Active listening, empathy, and successful communication are examples of these abilities.

## Educational Assistance

Education is an important component of the lives of teens and young adults with ADHD, and particular educational help is frequently required.

## Individualized Education Plan (IEP) and 504 Plan

Individuals with impairments Education Act (IDEA) in the United States allows for the development of an Individualised Education Plan (IEP) for students with impairments, including ADHD. An IEP specifies specific accommodations and changes that will assist pupils in succeeding in school. It can include extra time on tests, special seating, and additional help with organizational and study skills.

A 504 Plan is another option for ADHD students. It is less thorough than an IEP, but it still includes adjustments to meet a student's learning requirements.

## College and University Accommodations

Teens with ADHD who are planning to attend college or university should look into the accommodations and support services that are available at their prefered institutions. These can include extra test-taking time, note-taking aid, and easily accessible organizational and time-management resources.

## Complementary and Alternative Approaches

Some people with ADHD and their families look into complementary and alternative therapies in addition to pharmacological and behavioral interventions. These can be used in conjunction with conventional treatments or on their own. It is critical to proceed with caution and to check with healthcare specialists.

## Nutrition and Exercise

Regular physical activity and a well-balanced diet can help reduce ADHD symptoms. Exercise promotes the release of neurotransmitters such as dopamine and norepinephrine, which can improve concentration and mood. Proper diet ensures that the body gets the nutrients it needs, which might affect brain function.

## Meditation and mindfulness

Mindfulness practices, such as meditation and yoga, can help people with ADHD become more self-aware, manage stress, and focus better. These practices encourage people to be present in the moment, which is a useful ability for dealing with impulsivity and distractions.

## Supplements and Dietary Strategies

Some people look at dietary changes and supplements as alternatives to ADHD medication. Omega-3 fatty acids, for example, have been researched for their possible help in symptom reduction. However, before making large dietary changes or using supplements, it is critical to check with a healthcare expert.

## Neurofeedback and Biofeedback

Neurofeedback and biofeedback are therapeutic treatments that educate people how to control their brain activity and physiological responses. Although their effectiveness varies from person to person, these approaches can enhance attention and impulse control.

It is crucial to approach complementary and alternative approaches with a critical yet open attitude. What works for one person may not work for another, and the evidence for alternative procedures may be weaker than for conventional treatments.

There is no one-size-fits-all method for addressing ADHD in teens and young adults. Treatments tailored to an individual's specific needs are frequently used in effective management. Individuals with ADHD and their families can thrive not despite, but because of, ADHD by exploring medication management, behavioural therapies, educational support, and complementary approaches.

## Inspirational Story

*Sarah was a bright and creative 15-year-old once upon a time. Sarah was a tornado of ideas and enthusiasm, but she struggled to focus on studies and finish projects. Her room was a treasure trove of* artistic undertakings, but her organising abilities were lacking. Sarah's parents were becoming increasingly concerned about her academic performance and her dwindling confidence.

## Medication Management: A Fresh Start

*Sarah's parents felt that it was time to seek expert assistance. Sarah was diagnosed with ADHD after visiting with a child psychiatrist and undergoing a full evaluation. Her parents, who were first sceptical about medicine, decided to give it a shot, believing it could be a useful tool in her ADHD management.*

*Sarah was administered a low amount of a stimulant medicine, and they began the medication management journey. It wasn't an overnight change, but as they worked tirelessly with their healthcare professional to fine-tune the dosage and handle any side effects, they began to observe major changes.*

# Chapter 4

# Parenting Strategies

Parenting an ADHD adolescent or young adult can be both gratifying and hard. It is critical to provide a supporting and nurturing atmosphere in which they can grow. In this chapter, we'll look at different parenting practices to assist you negotiate the unique challenge of raising an ADHD child.

## Creating a Supportive Environment

A supportive atmosphere is essential for effective parenting of an ADHD child. It serves as the foundation for their development, learning, and overall well-being. Here are some ideas for how to create such an environment:

# How to Understand ADHD

Begin by learning more about ADHD. The first step in providing appropriate support is to understand the ailment, its symptoms, and its impact on daily life. Knowledge enables you to be more patient, sympathetic, and responsive to the needs of your child.

## Consistency and Structure

Structured environments are typically beneficial to children with ADHD. Set up routines for daily activities such as bedtime, homework, and mealtimes. Predictable timetables can assist your youngster in managing their time and decreasing anxiety.

## Setting reasonable expectations

Establish age-appropriate, attainable goals for your child. Recognise that they may want extra time and assistance to complete activities, so be patient and empathetic when they face difficulties.

## Positive Reinforcement

Recognise and appreciate your child's efforts and accomplishments by using positive reinforcement. Praise their accomplishments, no matter how minor, and offer rewards for completing tasks or demonstrating excellent conduct.

## Order and Organisation

Assist your child in becoming more organized. Teach them how to use organizing tools such as calendars, to-do lists, and organizational apps. Establish a homework area and aid them in keeping their own space tidy.

## Stress Reduction

Teach your youngster stress-reduction skills like deep breathing exercises or mindfulness practises. These abilities can assist them in dealing with the emotional ups and downs that are common with ADHD.

## Conflict Resolution and Communication

Effective communication is essential in every parent-child relationship, but it is especially critical when raising an ADHD child. Here's how to communicate effectively and settle conflicts:

- **Listening Actively**: Active listening should be practiced. Give your complete attention to your child when they speak, and ask questions to ensure you grasp their point of view.

- **Open Discussion**: Make a conversational environment that is open and non-judgmental. Encourage your child to express their feelings and views, and to listen to their concerns.

- **Dispute Resolution**: When disagreements develop, concentrate on working together to find solutions. Collaborative problem-solving allows your child to accept responsibility for their actions and develops critical decision-making abilities.

- **Use "I" statements**: When explaining a subject, use "I" phrases to express your feelings and concerns. stating "You never finish your work," for instance, might be preferable than stating "I am concerned when you do not complete your assignments."

- **Avoid Blame**: Avoid blaming your child for ADHD-related difficulties. Remember that their behavior is a result of their condition, not a decision.

- **Set Boundaries**: Define the rules and boundaries clearly. Your consistency in expectations assists your child in understanding the repercussions of their behavior.

## Building Self-Esteem

Building your child's self-esteem is critical for navigating the obstacles of ADHD. A high feeling of self-worth can help them handle challenges with confidence. Here's how you can help them feel better about themselves:

- **Celebrate Achievements:** Recognise and appreciate your child's accomplishments, no matter how minor. Encourage kids to be proud of their accomplishments, whether it's a well-done project or a personal achievement.
- **Highlight Strengths**: Highlight your child's abilities and capabilities. Recognising their unique abilities and

skills can boost self-esteem and motivation.

- **Focus on Effort**: Encourage your child to concentrate on their efforts rather than the end result. Remind yourself that perseverance and hard work are more vital than rapid achievement.

- **Positive Affirmations**: Provide positive reinforcement and reassurance. Tell your youngster that you believe in them and that they are capable of conquering obstacles.

- **Promote Independence:** Assist your child in gaining independence. Encourage them to take on tasks and make decisions so that they can gain confidence.
- **Offer Encouragement:** Be a source of inspiration. Remind your child that you are there to assist them and that

setbacks are a normal part of growth and learning.

## Inspirational Story

*Follow Sarah, a 16-year-old girl with ADHD, as she navigates life with the help of her parents, Lisa and John.*

### *Creating a Supportive Environment*

*Sarah's parents have always been confident in her abilities. They recognised that she faced particular obstacles as a result of her ADHD, but they never allowed it to define her. They began their adventure by learning everything they could about ADHD, attending courses, and joining support groups. This information aided them in creating a welcoming workplace.*

*Consistency was essential. Emma followed a daily schedule that included schoolwork, housework, and downtime. Knowing what to expect made her feel less anxious and* more in control. Every morning, Emma's parents would go through her daily plan, ensuring she knew what was expected of her and had all the resources she need.

Setting reasonable expectations was a critical component of their strategy. Lisa and John saw that Emma needs more time and assistance with things. Instead than putting pressure on her to be flawless, they encouraged and commended her attempts. It wasn't so much about the grade as it was about the work she put in.

Positive reinforcement was a big deal in their house. Emma was praised and encouraged for all her modest and large accomplishments. Her parents praised her accomplishments, which boosted her self-esteem.

Emma's room, which was formerly crowded and chaotic, was transformed into an arranged haven. She learnt how to use calendars and to-do lists properly with the *help of her parents. Her desk had become her haven, and she enjoyed managing her chores.*

*Emma's parents also taught her how to deal with stress. They did mindfulness and relaxation techniques together, giving Emma tools to help her control her emotions. She learned to accept her energy and channel it into useful endeavours.*

## Conflict Resolution and Communication

*Emma and her parents have a close relationship based on open communication. During their interactions, they engaged in active listening. Emma knew her parents would be open to discussing any topic or sharing her feelings.*
*During disagreements, they concentrated on working together to find solutions. Instead of condemning or blaming one another, they worked together to solve*

*problems. Emma was able to develop responsibility and good decision-making skills as a result of this method.*

*It was normal practise in their household to employ "I" statements. Instead of stating, "You never finish your assignments," Emma's parents would reply, "I'm worried when you don't finish your work," which kept their communication productive and non-confrontational.*

### Self-Esteem Development

*Emma's self-esteem grew thanks to her parents' supervision. They acknowledged her accomplishments, whether it was completing a job on time or finally learning to ride a bike. Emma was extremely proud of her accomplishments, no matter how minor.*

*Her parents frequently emphasized her strengths. Emma was a talented artist, and her parents made sure she had the time and resources she needed to develop her skills. They applauded her ingenuity and loved her artwork, which boosted her self-esteem.*

*Emma learnt to value work over results. Her parents encouraged her to do her best and stressed the importance of progress above perfection. This attitude assisted her in overcoming setbacks and problems.*

*Positive affirmations were part of my everyday routine. Her parents continually told her that she could achieve everything she set her mind to. They believed in her abilities and made certain she was aware of them.*

*Another tenet of their strategy was independence. Emma rapidly increased her duties, from schoolwork to managing her daily calendar. This independence aided her in developing self-esteem.*

*Emma's parents were her greatest source of support. They told her that they would be there for her through the highs and lows. Emma felt she could rely on them, and their consistent support helped to build her self-esteem.*

*Emma's journey continued as she accepted her individuality and the obstacles that came with ADHD. She excelled in her organized, supportive environment, thanks to her parents' dedication and affection. Emma earned the confidence to face life's obstacles front on through efficient communication and a focus on self-esteem building. Her parents' parenting skills not only assisted her in coping with ADHD, but also allowed her to grow in her own unique way.*

You may create a supportive atmosphere for your child to thrive despite their ADHD by applying these parenting practices. Remember that parenting is an ongoing process, and your assistance can have a significant impact on your child's life. Effective communication, consistency, and self-esteem boosting are all great tools for parents to use as they negotiate the specific problems and strengths that come with ADHD in teenagers and young adults.

# Chapter 5

# School and Academic Support

In this chapter, we'll look at school and academic help for ADHD teens and young adults. Education is an important element of their life, and understanding how to navigate the educational system is critical to their success. We'll look at Individualised Education Plans (IEPs) and 504 Plans, as well as study skills, time management, and communicating with teachers and school personnel.

## Individualized Education Plans (IEPs) and 504 Plans

# Understanding Individualised Education Programmes (IEPs) and 504 Plans

Individualised Education Plans (IEPs) and 504 Plans are specific tools used to provide academic support and accommodations to students with impairments such as ADHD. They differ greatly from one another even if they share certain characteristics..

## IEPs (Individualized Education Plans)

IEPs are comprehensive plans designed expressly for students who face substantial academic challenges as a result of their disability. A student's handicap must have a significant impact on their ability to access the general education curriculum in order to qualify for an IEP.

IEPs usually include specific goals and objectives, as well as specialised instruction and accompanying services such as speech therapy or occupational therapy. They are legally enforceable and offer significant support to kids, ensuring they obtain the services they need to flourish academically.

## 504 Plans

Section 504 Plans, called after Section 504 of the Rehabilitation Act, are intended to accommodate students with impairments. A student must have a disability that significantly limits one or more major living activities, including learning, to be eligible for a 504 Plan.

While 504 Plans do not provide the same degree of specialized instruction as IEPs, they do provide children with accommodations and adjustments to assist them access the general education curriculum. This can include extra test time, prefered sitting, and the use of assistive technology.

## Obtaining an IEP or 504 Plan

The first step in acquiring an IEP or 504 plan for your child with ADHD is to request an evaluation through your child's school. This evaluation will evaluate whether they qualify for one of these plans based on their educational needs.

During this process, it is critical to collaborate closely with school personnel. To establish the best solution, the school will undertake assessments and consult with teachers and parents.

## Key Components of an IEP or 504 Plan

When your child is eligible for an IEP or 504 plan, you will collaborate with the school to create a plan that meets their specific needs. These plans' key components may include:

- **Specific accommodations:** a description of the modifications and supports that your kid will receive in the classroom.

- **Goals and objectives:** setting educational goals and quantifiable targets that will assist your child in progressing.

- **Services and modifications:** a description of the services, specialist instruction, and any curricular changes that are required.

- **Timelines and review dates**: Establishing a timeline for plan implementation and conducting regular reviews to ensure its effectiveness.

- **Parental involvement:** Parental involvement entails encouraging your active participation in the development and monitoring of the strategy.

- **Transition planning:** addressing future needs, particularly if your child is facing a transition, such as the move from middle to high school.

## Study Skills and Time Management

Effective Study Techniques: Teaching your teen or young adult excellent study methods can improve their academic performance significantly. Here are some pointers:

- **Clean, Clutter-Free Workspace**: Assist your child in creating a clean, clutter-free workspace so they can focus without interruptions.

- **Note-Taking Strategies:** Encourage them to take orderly and succinct notes during lectures or when reading. Highlighting important areas and utilising colour coding can be beneficial.

- **Time Management:** Teach your youngster to manage their time efficiently by developing schedules and to-do lists. Setting defined priorities and goals for each study session helps enhance productivity.

- **Active Learning:** Encourage students to use active learning approaches such as summarising material in their own words, debating themes with peers, and making flashcards

- **Self-Testing**: Encourage self-quizzing and self-testing as useful methods of reinforcing learning and measuring comprehension.

- **Breaks and Rewards**: Encourage your child to take regular pauses to avoid burnout and to reward themselves when they hit goals in their study sessions.

# Time Management Strategies

Time management is an essential skill for ADHD students. Here are some suggestions to assist your child improve their time management:

a. **Use Digital Tools:** Assist your child in using digital tools on their smartphones or laptops, such as calendars, task management applications, and reminders.

b. **Prioritize Tasks**: Teach them to identify and prioritize high-priority tasks. Breaking down larger activities into smaller, more manageable chunks can also be beneficial.

c. **Set Realistic Goals**: Make sure your child sets reasonable daily and weekly goals that take into account their workload and deadlines.

d. **Create Routines:** Assist them in developing a daily schedule that includes devoted study time, housework, and relaxation. Consistency is essential.

e. **Reduce Distractions:** Inform them that they should reduce distractions by choosing a peaceful, clutter-free workspace and turning off unneeded notifications.

f. **Time Tracking**: Encourage your child to log their time in order to determine how they are spending it and make any required changes.

## Collaborating with Teachers and School Staff

Collaboration with teachers and school staff is critical to your child's academic success. Here's how to create a fruitful collaboration:

a. **Open Communication**: Maintain open lines of contact with teachers and school personnel. Share your child's diagnosis, any relevant documentation, and your support expectations.

b. **Regular Check-Ins:** Schedule regular check-ins with teachers to review your child's progress and any concerns. These sessions can aid in the timely resolution of difficulties.

c. **Understand Their Point of View**: Be open to understanding the teacher's point of view and the difficulties they face when managing a diverse classroom.

d. **Ask for Feedback:** Ask teachers for input on your child's behavior, performance, and any potential issues. This conversation might help you personalize support to your child's specific needs.

e. **Collaborative Problem Solving:** Approach any challenges or conflicts together. Collaborate with instructors to identify solutions that are beneficial to your child.

f. **Stay Informed:** Stay up to date on school policies, programmes, and resources for students with ADHD. This understanding enables you to effectively advocate for your child.

g. **Promote Accommodations**: If your kid has an IEP or 504 plan, make sure teachers are aware of the accommodations and modifications that should be provided in the classroom.

h. **Cultivate a Positive Relationship:** Fostering a positive relationship with teachers can result in a more supportive and inclusive learning environment for your child.

Navigating the educational world for your child with ADHD may seem daunting, but with the appropriate tactics and collaboration, you can help them excel academically. Understanding the subtleties of IEPs and 504 Plans, teaching effective study skills and time management, and cultivating a solid partnership with teachers and school personnel are critical in providing your kid with the academic help he or she requires to achieve.

## Inspirational Story

### *Academic and School Support—Sarah's Triumph*

*Let's look at Sarah's life and her school path, highlighting the academic support measures that changed her experience.*

### *Sarah's Academic Difficulties*

*Sarah was a brilliant, imaginative 14-year-old with an insatiable desire to study. Her life, however, was distinguished by continual academic struggles as a result of her ADHD. Simple activities that most students found doable, such as paying attention in class or staying organized, appeared impossible to her.*

### *The Implementation of an IEP*

*Sarah's parents saw the difficulties their daughter was experiencing and chose to look into academic support possibilities. They collaborated closely with her school to begin the process of preparing an IEP (individualized education plan).*

*Sarah's IEP included modifications such as extra test time, a quiet room for assignments, and the use of assistive technology to assist her with note-taking. These changes enabled her to properly access the curriculum, considerably lessening her anxiety.*

# Time Management and Study Skills

Sarah's parents recognised the need for strong study skills and time management for her success. They introduced her to various strategies, including:

- **Organized Workspace**: They updated her study area together. Her workstation became a productive haven, free of interruptions and clutter.

- **Note-Taking Techniques**: During lessons, they taught Sarah how to take brief, ordered notes. She became more efficient in capturing important information by using color-coding and summarizing key points.

- **Time Management:** Sarah and her parents worked together to develop a daily routine and to-do list. Setting priorities and specific goals for each study session became second nature.

- *Active Learning:* *They urged her to take an active role in her education. Sarah began summarizing her studies in her own words, discussing themes with her peers, and making flashcards to help her remember.*

- *Breaks and Rewards: They recognised the importance of taking breaks in order to avoid burnout. Sarah learnt to create goals for herself and reward herself when she met them during her study sessions.*

## Partnership with Teachers and School Personnel

*Sarah's success was built on her ability to maintain positive relationships with teachers and school personnel.*

*Sarah's parents kept open lines of communication open with her teachers.*

*They discussed her ADHD diagnosis and supplied pertinent papers to ensure that everyone was aware of her specific needs.*

*Regular check-ins with teachers allowed for discussions about Sarah's progress and any concerns. This open conversation aided in the rapid resolution of issues and modifications.*

*Sarah's parents recognised the difficulties teachers encounter while managing a diverse classroom. They attempted to comprehend the teacher's point of view and collaborated to create the best learning environment for Sarah.*

***Collaborative Problem-Solving:*** *When problems or disagreements developed, Sarah's parents used a collaborative method to resolve them. Working in tandem with teachers, they found solutions that were mutually beneficial.*

*Staying Informed:* *They took the initiative to learn about school policies, programmes, and resources for children with ADHD. Their knowledge enabled them to effectively advocate for Sarah.*

## Sarah's Victory

*Sarah's life improved once she implemented these academic support measures. Her problems converted into chances for growth. She not only conquered her scholastic barriers but began to flourish in her academics.*

*The combination of her IEP, effective study skills, and time management, along with the collaborative support of her teachers and school staff, unlocked her potential. Sarah's journey with ADHD became a testimonial to the power of academic support in enabling kids to not only overcome problems but to thrive in their scholastic aspirations.*

*The determination and dedication of Sarah's parents, together with the supporting environment created by her school, turned her scholastic problems into a victory. She learned not only to manage her ADHD but to embrace it as a unique part of herself, equipping her with the resilience and skills to conquer any academic endeavor.*

# Chapter 6

# Lifestyle and Self-Care

In this chapter, we will look at the important areas of lifestyle and self-care that have a big impact on the well-being of ADHD teens and young adults. These aspects, which range from diet and nutrition to exercise, physical health, and stress management techniques, all play an important part in assisting people with ADHD to live satisfying lives.

## Diet and Nutrition

A healthy diet and sufficient nutrition are important for everyone, but they are especially important for those with ADHD. In this section, we'll talk about the significance of diet in controlling ADHD symptoms and promoting general health.

# The Relationship Between Diet and ADHD

While nutrition cannot "cure" ADHD, it can have an impact on the severity of symptoms and overall well-being. Specific dietary components have been demonstrated in studies to either increase or treat ADHD symptoms. Here are some important considerations:

- **Omega-3 Fatty Acids**: Omega-3 fatty acids, which are abundant in fish, flaxseeds, and walnuts, have been linked to better cognitive performance and attentiveness. Incorporating these foods into your diet can be advantageous.

- **Protein**: Protein-rich foods, such as lean meats, beans, and lentils, give a consistent release of energy and can aid in mood and focus stabilization.

- **Complex Carbohydrates**: Complex carbs, such as whole grains and vegetables, slowly release glucose into the bloodstream, which can help maintain consistent energy levels and mood.

- **Sugar and Artificial Additives:** According to several research, too much sugar and artificial additives in processed foods may aggravate ADHD symptoms in certain people. Reducing your consumption of sugary snacks and food dyes can be beneficial.

- **Hydration**: Concentration and focus can be affected by dehydration. Keeping hydrated is critical for proper brain function.

# Practical Dietary Suggestions

Here are some helpful hints to help people with ADHD keep a healthy diet:

- **Regular Meals**: Encourage regular meals and snacks to keep blood sugar levels steady.

- **Hydration**: Make sure your teen drinks enough of water throughout the day.

- **Reduce Processed Foods:** Limit your intake of highly processed foods, which are generally heavy in sugar and artificial additives.

- **Omega-3 Rich Foods**: Include omega-3 fatty acid sources such as salmon, chia seeds, and flaxseeds in your diet.

- **Whole Grain Ingredients:** In your child's diet, choose whole grains over refined grains.

- **Variety**: Encourage the consumption of a variety of fruits and vegetables to obtain necessary vitamins and minerals.

## Physical Fitness and Exercise

Physical fitness and exercise are critical in treating ADHD symptoms. Frequent exercise has been shown to enhance mood, focus, and general wellbeing.

## The Advantages of Exercise for ADHD

Exercise has a number of advantages for those with ADHD.

- **Improved Focus:** Physical activity can boost the release of neurotransmitters associated with attention and focus, such as dopamine and norepinephrine.

- **Reducing Stress:** Exercise relieves tension and anxiety, which are major problems for people with ADHD.

- **More Restful Sleep:** Regular exercise can lead to better sleep quality, which is important in managing ADHD symptoms.

- **Enhanced Executive Function**: It has been proven that physical activity improves executive functions such as organisation, time management, and task initiation.

- **Increased Self-Esteem:** Physical goals achieved through exercise can enhance self-esteem and confidence.

# How to Fit Exercise Into Your Everyday Routine

Here are some ideas for working fitness into your regular routine:

- **Find Activities They Enjoy:** Encourage your youngster to try out different physical activities to see what they like. Dance and team sports, as well as yoga and martial arts, are all possibilities.

- **Set Realistic Goals**: Assist your youngster in setting attainable fitness goals. Begin with simple, manageable goals, gradually increasing the intensity and time.

- **Consistency is important:** Intensity is less crucial than consistency. Even brief bouts of exercise on a regular basis can be beneficial.

- **Have Some Fun**: Exercise does not have to be difficult. Involve the entire family or incorporate games and challenges to make it more enjoyable.

- **Create a Routine:** Create a regular exercise routine. Consistency aids in the formation of an exercise habit.

# Techniques for Stress Management and Relaxation

Stress management is critical for people with ADHD since it can increase symptoms and damage overall well-being. Teaching stress management and relaxation techniques has the potential to influence the game.

# The Importance of Stress Management

Individuals with ADHD can be affected by stress in a variety of ways:

a. **Focus and Attention**: High stress levels might make it difficult to concentrate.

b. **Emotional Control:** Emotional reactivity and mood swings can be exacerbated by stress.

c. **Frustration**: Stress can cause procrastination and difficulties starting work.

d. **Physical Signs and Symptoms:** Physical manifestations of stress include tension and agitation.

# Stress Reduction Techniques

Here are some stress management and relaxation practices that teens and young adults with ADHD might benefit from:

- **Mindfulness Meditation:** Meditation and deep breathing are two mindfulness strategies that can help people stay grounded and minimize worry.

- **Exercise**: Physical activity on a regular basis is an effective stress reliever.

- **Time Management:** Teach excellent time management strategies to assist lessen the stress of approaching deadlines.

- **Creative Channels:** Encourage the use of creative activities such as art, music, or writing to express and control emotions.

- **Organization Skills:** Improve your organizational skills to help alleviate stress caused by disorganization.

- **Positive Self-Talk:** Encourage positive self-talk and self-compassion as stress-management skills.

- **Establishing a Routine:** Routines and timetables that are consistent can help to lessen uncertainty and stress.

Diet and nutrition, exercise, and stress management practices can have a significant impact on the well-being of teens and young adults with ADHD. These measures can assist individuals in managing their symptoms, improving their general health, and improving their quality of life.

# Inspirational Story

## *Sarah's Transformation: Lifestyle and Self-Care*

*Let's go on a trip with Sarah, an 18-year-old with ADHD, to see how lifestyle and self-care practices impacted her life.*

### *Sarah's Dietary Change*

*Sarah's life was a tornado of creativity and activity, but her ADHD frequently made her daily routine difficult. Her family decided to make some modifications after realizing the potential impact of her diet on her symptoms.*

*They changed her eating habits, adding omega-3 fatty acid-rich foods like salmon and flaxseeds. These changes appeared to give her more steady cognitive function and a longer attention span.*

*Her family also worked hard to limit her intake of processed foods heavy in sugar* and other additives. Sugary snacks were replaced with healthy alternatives, and food labels were thoroughly scrutinized for dangerous colors and ingredients.

To stay hydrated, Sarah began drinking more water throughout the day. Proper hydration enabled her to maintain consistent energy levels and mood, which had a big impact on her general well-being.

While these dietary adjustments did not "cure" her ADHD, they did make her life more liveable and aid in the management of her symptoms.

## Sarah's Journey to a Healthier Way of Life

Sarah's life was transformed by regular exercise, which had a substantial impact on her ADHD symptoms. It became an effective tool for controlling her focus, mood, and energy levels.

Sarah fell in love with yoga. The practise gave not only physical activity but also stress relief and relaxation. She increased her focus, emotional stability, and self-esteem as a result of her yoga practise.

Her family helped her create reasonable exercise objectives. They highlighted the value of fun and the benefits of regular physical activity above high intensity. Short, frequent sessions became a vital part of her everyday life, and consistency became a key value.

## Stress Reduction and Relaxation Methods

Sarah's life with ADHD had often been defined by stress. She was frequently overwhelmed by the pressures of school, social interactions, and symptom management. Her family introduced her to stress management and relaxation *techniques because they recognised the importance of teaching these skills.*

*Sarah discovered mindfulness meditation and deep breathing exercises. These techniques assisted her in remaining grounded and reducing anxiety. Taking a few moments to pause and breathe deeply became her way of finding calm in the midst of chaos whenever she felt overwhelmed or stressed.*

*Incorporating exercise into her daily routine was critical to stress management. Physical activity provided a healthy outlet for her emotions and a respite from the academic and social pressures she was subjected to.*

*Sarah also used creative activities like writing and painting to express herself and cope with stress. These creative outlets allowed her to express herself and release pent-up emotions.*

*Working on her organizational skills was an important part of Sarah's stress management strategy. Her ability to stay organized not only aided her academic performance but also reduced the anxiety associated with disorganization.*

*Sarah found comfort in her routines and schedules, which provided predictability in her often unpredictable world.*

*Sarah's life was transformed after she implemented these lifestyle and self-care strategies. While her ADHD remained a part of her life, she learned the tools and resilience she needed to manage her symptoms and live a happy life. Her ADHD journey became a path of self-discovery and personal growth when she combined a balanced diet, regular exercise, and effective stress management skills. Sarah learnt to thrive despite her disability, demonstrating the incredible power of lifestyle and self-care in the lives of teens and young adults with ADHD.*

# Chapter 7

# Transitioning to Adulthood

Transitioning from youth to adulthood is an important milestone for every young person. For those with ADHD, this adjustment can come with special problems and implications. In this chapter, we will look at how to prepare for college or work, how to acquire independent living skills, and how to comprehend legal and financial issues as young adults with ADHD embark on their journey to independence.

## Preparing for College or Work

The move to college or the workforce is a key stage in the life of a young adult with ADHD. This section will go over how to successfully prepare for this shift.

# College or Work: A Personal Choice

One of the first decisions is whether to pursue higher education, enter the workforce, or engage in a combination of both. This is a highly personal decision that should reflect an individual's abilities, interests, and career ambitions. It is critical to remember the following:

- **Career Goals:** Consider your interests and career goals. How does your ADHD affect your chosen career path?

- **Higher Education:** If you intend to attend college, look for universities that offer ADHD-supportive services.

- **Entry into the Workforce**: If you're going straight to work, look at companies that provide inclusive work environments.

# Organizing for Success

Regardless of the path selected, organization is essential. Here are a few ideas:

- **Time Management**: Improve your time management abilities, whether for class or work deadlines. Consider tools such as calendars and planners.

- **Create a productive study and working environment**: Reduce distractions, provide appropriate illumination, and have all necessary equipment on hand.

- **Effective Communication**: Learn how to effectively explain your needs to academics, employers, and colleagues. Discuss any accommodations or techniques that will help you succeed.

- **Study or Work Habits**: Establish good study or work habits. Understand and use your best learning style and work habits to your benefit.

## Independent Living Skills

Individuals with ADHD must learn independent living skills as part of their journey to maturity.

## Self-Care and Daily Life

Managing daily life independently necessitates self-care, which includes:

- **Healthcare**: Understand your healthcare needs and how to obtain medical services.

- **Nutrition**: Learn to plan and prepare healthy meals while taking dietary needs into account.

- **Personal Hygiene:** Establish daily personal hygiene practices.

- **Household Chores**: Practice keeping a clean living environment and managing home duties.

## Financial Literacy

Another important part of independent living is financial management:

- **Budgeting**: Discover how to develop and manage a budget while tracking income and expenses.

- **Banking**: Understand financial services, such as checking and savings accounts, as well as good money management.

- **Savings and investments:** Consider saving for the future and investing when appropriate.

- **Debt Management**: Understand how to manage debts such as credit cards and loans.

## Transportation and Mobility

It is critical to be mobile and to have reliable transportation:

- **Driving**: If you must drive, learn about road safety, rules, and upkeep.

- **Public Transportation:** Understand how to use public transportation.

- **Navigational Skills**: Practice finding your way around using maps or GPS.

## Legal and Financial Considerations

For young adults with ADHD, navigating the legal and financial aspects of adulthood is critical. The following are some points to consider:

## Legal Issues

- **Legal Rights:** As an adult, be aware of your legal rights. This includes the ability to vote, sign contracts, and make your own healthcare decisions.

- **Legal Documents**: Depending on your needs and circumstances, consider creating legal documents such as a power of attorney or health care proxy.

- **Accommodations**: If necessary, ensure that you have access to any legal accommodations that will help you succeed in college or at work.

## Financial Considerations

- **Income and Taxes**: Understand the operation of income taxes, including deductions and credits.

- **Insurance**: Learn about the various forms of insurance available, such as health, vehicle, and renter's insurance, and how they work.

- **Savings and Investments**: Consider your savings and investing possibilities, as well as the implications for taxes and financial stability.

- **Debt Management**: Learn how to effectively manage debts in order to maintain good financial health.

- **Credit Scores**: Understand the significance of credit scores and how to build and maintain good credit.

Navigating the transition to adulthood requires a thoughtful approach, particularly for young adults with ADHD. Preparing for college or work, mastering independent living skills, and understanding legal and financial considerations are essential steps towards achieving independence and success. These abilities and insights enable people with ADHD to face the challenges and opportunities of adulthood with confidence and readiness.

# Inspirational Story

### Sarah's Journey Through Adulthood

*Sarah had always been determined and motivated. Her ADHD, while posing unique hurdles, didn't stop her from her dreams of obtaining further education and gaining independence. As she launched on her road to adulthood, she faced key decisions and learned essential abilities to manage this transitional era.*

### Preparing for College or Work
*For Sarah, the choice was clear—she aspired to attend college and was*

*passionate about pursuing a career in psychology. She was aware, however, that her journey would necessitate careful planning and effective strategies:*

- ***Career Goals:** Sarah reflected on her career goals, taking into account her interest in psychology and her ADHD. She recognised that her condition provided her with unique insights and empathy, which could be useful in her future career.*

- ***Organizing for Success:** Sarah developed robust time management skills. She employed digital tools to maintain a well-structured calendar, ensuring she never missed a lesson or an assignment due. She learned how to create an optimal study environment free from distractions by investing in noise-canceling headphones and adopting productive study habits.*

- ***Effective Communication:*** *Sarah understood the value of effective communication. She didn't hesitate to talk to her professors about her ADHD and the accommodations she needed. This discussion resulted in extra time for exams and advance access to lecture notes.*

## Skills for Independent Living

*Learning to live alone became an important element of Sarah's road to adulthood.*

***Self-Care and Daily Life:*** *Sarah learned how to handle her healthcare requirements, schedule visits, and refill prescriptions. She learned skills for keeping her living area and established a regular routine for personal hygiene.*
- ***Financial Literacy:*** *Sarah addressed financial literacy by*

developing and sticking to a budget. She recognised the need of saving for the future and made monthly deposits to her savings account. She also learnt how to manage her credit wisely.

- **Transportation and Mobility:** Sarah earned her driver's license, becoming adept in road safety and car maintenance. She was at ease with public transit and had good navigation abilities.

## Legal and Financial Considerations

As an adult, Sarah accepted the legal and financial sides of her new existence.

- **Legal Concerns:** She was aware of her legal rights, such as the ability to vote and make healthcare decisions. Although she didn't require a power of attorney or a healthcare proxy, she was familiar with these forms.

- ***Financial Considerations****: Sarah was aware of her tax duties and filed them on time each year. She had health insurance through her employment and was also insured for her car. She managed her credit properly, keeping her credit score good.*

*Sarah's path to adulthood was exceptional. Her persistence, along with thorough preparation, enabled her to follow her ambitions of higher education and a rewarding profession. She was able to handle this changeover period with confidence and elegance after mastering independent living skills and comprehending legal and financial considerations. Sarah's tale demonstrated the possibilities of people with ADHD as they enter adulthood with determination and the correct abilities.*

# Chapter 8

# Social Relationships

Navigating the intricate landscape of social connections can be both gratifying and difficult, particularly for ADHD teens and young adults. In this chapter, we'll look at how to make friends and socialize, how to navigate dating and love relationships, and how to deal with peer pressure properly.

## Developing Social and Friendship Skills

Healthy friendships are essential for social well-being. Individuals with ADHD must hone their social skills in order to create and sustain these interactions.

### Making Friendships

Creating true friendships takes time and effort. Here are some important strategies:

- **Be true to yourself**: Authenticity is essential. Be yourself and let your own qualities come through. You are valued for who you are by true friends.

- **Shared Interests**: Look for people who share your interests and passions. Shared interests or activities can provide a solid basis for friendships.

- **Active Listening**: Maintaining eye contact, nodding, and asking follow-up questions are all examples of active listening. Demonstrate genuine attention in what people are saying.

- **Create the first contact:** Take the effort to create plans and contact pals. Others may be waiting for you to take the first step at times.

- **Maintain Boundaries:** Be mindful of your own and your friends' boundaries. Observe each other's personal space and limits.

## Developing Social Skills

Improving your social skills can improve the quality of your relationships:

- **Eye Contact**: Maintain appropriate eye contact during conversations to show attention and interest.

- **Empathy**: Put yourself in the shoes of others and try to comprehend their feelings and viewpoints.

- **Body Language:** Pay attention to your body language and make sure it corresponds to the message you want to express.

- **Conversation Skills**: Improve your ability to initiate and sustain discussions. Pose open-ended enquiries and respond thoughtfully.

- **Conflict Resolution**: Learn effective conflict resolution tactics for dealing with challenges that may emerge in friendships.

## Dating and Romantic Relationships

Navigating the world of dating and romantic relationships can be both exciting and difficult, particularly for people with ADHD. Here's how to tackle this social aspect:

- **Good Dating Dynamics:** Trust, mutual respect, and good communication are the foundations of healthy dating dynamics. Take a look at the following:

- **Communication that is Honest and Open:** Honest and open communication is crucial. Discuss your ADHD and how it may be affecting your relationship.

- **Establishing Clear Boundaries:** Establish clear boundaries that respect both partners' needs and levels of comfort.

- **Respecting Differences:** Accept your and your partner's differences. Recognise that your distinct qualities can be assets in a partnership.

- **Handling Rejection**: Rejection is an inevitable aspect of the dating process. Learn how to deal with it and go on.

## Managing ADHD in Relationships

ADHD can have an impact on relationships, but it does not have to be a barrier. Here's how to handle it successfully:

- **Medication and Therapy**: If medication or therapy helps you control your ADHD symptoms, stick with it.

- **Time Management**: Improve your time management abilities to be on time and attentive during dates.

- **Organization**: Keep track of important events, anniversaries, and plans.

- **Effective Communication:** Communicate your demands and problems to your partner effectively. Mutual understanding is essential.

## Dealing with Peer Pressure

Peer pressure is a normal component of social life, but it can present special issues for those with ADHD. Here's how to do it successfully:

**Understanding Peer Pressure**

Peer pressure can take many forms, ranging from subtle effects to more blatant coercion. Recognise when it is at work:

- **Positive vs. Negative Peer Pressure:** Peer pressure is not always negative. It can be beneficial and promote personal development.

- **Recognising Negative Pressure:** Be aware of circumstances in which peer pressure may lead to dangerous or harmful decisions.

- **Learning to Say No:** Develop your assertiveness and capacity to say no when faced with negative peer pressure.

# Developing Resilience

Developing resilience in the face of peer pressure entails increasing your inner will and self-confidence:

- **Understand your beliefs**: Be aware of your essential beliefs and ideals. This will assist you in making judgements that are consistent with your views.

- **Seek Help**: Surround yourself with encouraging friends who respect your decisions and boundaries.

- **Practice Assertiveness**: Develop assertiveness skills so that you can express your opinions and feelings clearly and boldly.

- **Healthy Coping Mechanisms:** Learn healthy coping mechanisms to deal with stress and discomfort without succumbing to negative peer pressure.

Navigating social relationships, dating, and peer pressure may be a fluid and ever-changing experience. Individuals with ADHD can form meaningful relationships and lead fulfilling social lives by cultivating healthy friendships, honing social skills, and effectively dealing with peer pressure. Remember that your biggest strengths in the domain of social relationships are authenticity and self-confidence.

## Inspirational Story

### Sarah's Journey in Social Relationships

*Sarah, a lively and motivated young adult with ADHD, set out on a voyage through the perplexing world of social interactions, dating, and peer pressure. Her narrative exemplifies the difficulties and triumphs that people with ADHD might face in these areas.*

## Developing Social Skills and Friendships

Sarah was constantly eager to meet new people and make new acquaintances. She accepted the notion that having ADHD did not define her, but rather was one facet of her distinct personality. She used the following tactics to form deep friendships:

- **Authenticity**: Sarah recognised that her strength was her authenticity. She remained loyal to herself, allowing her eccentricities and strengths to emerge. Her distinct viewpoint and overwhelming energy drew individuals who valued her for who she was.

- Sarah joined a local art club, which fueled her enthusiasm for painting. She met like-minded people who shared her passion for creating. Their shared love of art served as the *foundation for deep and lasting friendships.*

- **Active Listening**: *Sarah used active listening to engage with people during conversations. She discovered that displaying real interest in her friends' life and experiences helped them feel appreciated and heard.*

- **Contact Initiation:** *Sarah recognised the need of taking the initiative. She didn't wait for people to arrange plans; instead, she asked friends to art classes, movie evenings, and coffee dates. Her initiative enriched her social life.*

- **Keeping limits:** *Sarah was conscious of her limits as she made new friends. She knew when to give her pals space and the value of personal boundaries.*

*Alongside building friendships, Sarah honed her social skills:*

- **Eye Contact**: *She made an attempt to keep eye contact during chats, demonstrating that she was totally engaged in the interaction.*

- **Empathy**: *Sarah practiced empathy by imagining herself in the shoes of her friends in order to better comprehend their emotions and views.*

- **Body Language**: *She was aware of her body language and made sure it matched the message she intended to express.*

- **Conversation Skills**: *Sarah improved her ability to initiate and sustain discussions. She posed open-ended questions and insightful* *responses, resulting in meaningful interactions.*

- ***Conflict Resolution:*** *Sarah developed excellent conflict resolution skills to address any conflicts that arose in her friendships from time to time. She discovered that having open and honest conversations resulted in better bonds.*

## Romantic Relationships and Dating

*Sarah's experience into the world of dating and romantic relationships was full of excitement and self-discovery. She tackled this part of her life by keeping the following concepts in mind:*

- ***Open and Honest Communication:*** *Honesty and openness were essential. Sarah was open about her ADHD and talked about how it would effect her relationship. Her spouse, Ben, valued* her candor and stood with her through any difficulties.

- **Understanding Boundaries:** It was critical to establish clear boundaries. Sarah and Ben talked about their personal boundaries and comfort zones, making sure both parties felt respected and protected.

- **Respecting Differences**: Sarah and Ben appreciated each other's differences. They recognised that their differences strengthened their relationship and made it more vibrant and fulfilling.

- **Handling Rejection:** Sarah, like everyone else, experienced rejection during her dating journey. She learnt to deal with it gracefully, considering it as an opportunity to grow and find a better fit.

## Managing Peer Pressure

*Sarah faced peer pressure in social situations, but her perseverance and self-assurance enabled her handle it successfully:*

- **Understanding Positive and Negative Peer Pressure:** *Sarah recognised the distinction between positive and negative peer pressure. She accepted her friends' good impacts that fostered personal growth and self-expression*

- **Identifying Negative Peer Pressure:** *Sarah was wary about negative peer pressure. She recognised when to avoid situations that could lead to unhealthy or unsafe decisions.*

- **Learning to Say No:** *Sarah honed her assertiveness skills by learning* *how to firmly say no when confronted with negative peer pressure. Her ability to set boundaries demonstrated her strength and self-assurance.*

- ***Developing Resilience:** Sarah developed resilience by first recognising her essential beliefs and ideals. She surrounded herself with people who supported her decisions and boundaries. When she was going through a tough time, she used healthy coping techniques including art, writing, and spending time with her supporting friends.*

*Sarah's journey through friendship, dating, and dealing with peer pressure demonstrated her resilience and self-assurance. Her open-hearted attitude to relationships and genuineness made her a beloved friend and partner. Sarah's experiences showed that people with ADHD* can form deep and enduring friendships, embrace romance, and resist harmful influences, ultimately prospering in the domain of social relationships.

# Chapter 9

# Resources and Support

We explore the essential tools and services that are accessible for adolescents and young adults with ADHD in this chapter. We will discuss the advantages of counseling and support groups, the function of online forums and applications, and where to go for licensed experts who can help and support you on your path.

## Support Groups and Counseling

There are some difficulties associated with having ADHD, but you don't have to confront them alone. Counseling and support groups may be very helpful for teenagers and young adults who need direction, understanding, and doable solutions.

# Support Groups

Support groups provide a secure environment where you may interact with others who understand what you're going through, acquire insights, and share experiences. This is why they are advantageous:

- **Understanding**: You will meet others in a support group who have comparable struggles. This comprehension may be reassuring as well as powerful.

- **Shared Strategies**: Members often exchange practical methods for handling ADHD, such as time management and organizing advice.

- **Emotional Support:** It's a safe space for you to vent your emotions and grievances. People who have been in your position before might provide you emotional support and encouragement.

- **Reduced Isolation**: Anxiety may sometimes result in feelings of loneliness. Support groups work against this by fostering a feeling of belonging and community.

**Counseling:** Cognitive-behavioral therapy (CBT), a kind of counseling, may provide individualized advice for handling the symptoms of ADHD and associated difficulties.

**Skills Development**: You may acquire important skills for time management, organization, and emotional control with the aid of counselors.

**Self-Acceptance**: Counseling may be very beneficial for teenagers and young adults who are having problems with their self-esteem since it fosters self-acceptance and self-compassion.

**Stress Management:** Handling stress is a big aspect of taking care of ADHD. Through counseling, you may learn stress-reduction strategies to keep your well being intact.

**Effective Strategies:** Cognitive behavioral therapy (CBT), for example, focuses on creating behavioral and cognitive strategies that enhance your day-to-day functioning.

## Online Communities and Apps

There are many tools and services available in the digital era that may help people with ADHD. When it comes to easily available aid, online groups and applications may be quite beneficial.

## Online Communities

Online forums devoted to ADHD provide a platform for communication and knowledge exchange:

- **Information Exchange**: You may ask questions and get assistance from a worldwide network of people who understand ADHD by using forums and discussion boards.

- **Success Stories**: It may be inspiring and uplifting to read about other people's struggles and victories.

- **Sharing of Resources:** Members often exchange useful resources, such as suggested books, practical tools, and applications.

- **24/7 Assistance**: With the 24/7 availability of online communities, you can always get the help and support you need.

## Apps and Tools

Digital technologies and mobile applications may be great partners in the management of ADHD:

- **Task Management**: By keeping track of your tasks and due dates, apps like Trello or Todoist assist you in maintaining organization.

- **Time Tracking**: You may increase productivity by keeping an eye on how you spend your time and using tools like RescueTime or Toggl.

- **Meditation and Mindfulness**: To help with stress management and attention enhancement, apps such as Calm and Headspace include guided mindfulness exercises and meditation.

- **Learning Support**: Engaging methods to enhance your knowledge and abilities may be found in apps like Khan Academy and Duolingo.

## Finding Qualified Professionals

Getting expert advice is essential to successfully controlling ADHD. Here's how to locate knowledgeable professionals that can provide you the assistance you need.

### Psychiatrists and Psychologists

- **Ask for Recommendations:** Start by contacting your primary care physician or other reliable people in your network for suggestions.

- **Check Credentials:** Check the qualifications and background of the experts you are thinking about hiring. Seek for qualified psychologists and psychiatrists with board certification.

- **Speak with Several Experts**: Never be afraid to seek advice from many professionals. It is crucial to get the correct fit.

## Counselors and therapists

- **Ask for Referrals:** Consult reliable sources for recommendations, same as you would while looking for psychologists and psychiatrists.

- **Specialization**: Seek for experts who focus on ADHD or similar disorders. They will comprehend your difficulties on a deeper level.

- **Therapeutic Approach**: A variety of therapeutic techniques may be used by different therapists. Pick the one that most closely matches your preferences and needs.

## Communities and support groups on the internet

- **Local Support Groups**: For information on nearby ADHD support groups, see your healthcare practitioner or go through local directories.

- **Online Communities**: Ask members of trustworthy online ADHD groups and forums who have had good experiences working with specialists for referrals.

An important first step on your path to successful ADHD treatment is getting in touch with experts in the field. Their knowledge might help you overcome obstacles by offering you specialized tactics and assistance.

In conclusion, teenagers and young adults with ADHD may benefit greatly from online forums, support groups, therapy, and digital technologies. These materials provide you with knowledge, tactics, and direction to help you properly manage your disease. Additionally, in order to get specialized assistance and knowledgeable direction on your path to a meaningful life, it is imperative that you locate experienced specialists that specialize in ADHD. Recall that there are experts and resources available to assist you at every stage of the process; you are not alone.

## Inspirational story

### Sarah's Journey to Empowerment: Resources and Support

*Sarah, a young lady with ADHD who is resourceful and motivated, set out on a quest to learn about the tools and resources that might help her deal with life's chances and problems.*

### Counseling and support groups

*Sarah realized she needed more specialized help when she entered her late teens in order to properly control her ADHD. She made the decision to look into therapy and support groups.*

### Support Groups

*Sarah discovered others who understood her struggles and experiences when she joined a local support group for ADHD. Here's what she discovered:*

- **Understanding Companions**: Sarah saw right away that this group of individuals understood her in a way that few others could. She felt less alone on her trip because of the supportive community.

- **Achievable Techniques:** Group members discussed useful techniques for managing ADHD. They spoke about time management, routine creation, and coping with emotional ups and downs. Sarah gained priceless knowledge that helped her live a more bearable everyday existence.

- **Emotional Resilience:** Sarah developed emotional resilience by venting her emotions and frustrations in a safe space. She found solace and optimism in the knowledge that other people had comparable difficulties.

- **Reduced Isolation**: She had sometimes felt alone because of her ADHD, but the support group turned into her safe refuge. She was able to fight those emotions of loneliness because of the relationships she created.

## Counseling

Sarah also went to therapy in order to improve her coping mechanisms. Working with an experienced therapist who was cognizant of ADHD, she encountered:

- **Development of Skills:** Sarah acquired crucial abilities for organizing her schedule, controlling her emotions, and managing her time via therapy. Her therapist provided tailored advice, which made it easier for her to put these techniques to use.

- **Awareness of Oneself:** Self-acceptance and self-compassion were encouraged throughout the therapy sessions. Sarah eventually started to consider her ADHD as a good characteristic that set her apart from the others.

- **Handling Stress**: In order to preserve her mental health despite the demands and difficulties of life, Sarah learned useful stress management skills.

- **Effective Strategies:** Sarah's therapist used cognitive-behavioral therapy (CBT) to assist her in creating useful behavioral and cognitive techniques. These techniques made her life better and gave her the strength to face obstacles head-on.

## Online Communities and Apps

Sarah has embraced applications and online networks in the digital era to improve her self-management abilities.

## Online Communities

Sarah joined a credible online group for ADHD and started contributing there. There, she discovered:

- **Information Sharing:** She had a place to ask questions and get advice from the community. She was able to get answers and ideas from a worldwide network of people who were knowledgeable about the complexities of ADHD.

- **Achievement Stories:** She was inspired by reading about the struggles and achievements of others. It served as a reminder that overcoming obstacles and achieving personal progress were possible.

- **Sharing of Resources:** Members contributed a multitude of materials, ranging from suggested reading lists and articles to practical tools and applications for everyday use.

- **24/7 Support:** The 24/7 availability of the online community guaranteed Sarah would always have access to help and information when she needed it.

## Tools and Apps

Sarah incorporated a number of digital tools and smartphone applications into her daily routine:

- **Management of Tasks:** She was able to maintain her organization and never miss a deadline thanks to apps like Trello and Todoist.

- **Time Monitoring:** She was able to increase productivity and keep an eye on her everyday activities thanks to tools like RescueTime and Toggl.

- **Mindfulness and Meditation:** With the use of apps like Calm and Headspace, which provide guided mindfulness exercises and meditation, Sarah is able to concentrate better and feel less stressed.

- **Education Assistance:** She found interesting methods to increase her knowledge and abilities using apps like Khan Academy and Duolingo.

## Identifying Eligible Experts

Sarah was determined to discover knowledgeable experts who could provide her with help, so she took action.

## Psychologists and psychiatrists

- Suggestions: She started by contacting her primary care physician for advice and trusted people in her network for recommendations.

- **Verification of Credentials:** Sarah made sure the specialists she was thinking about were qualified psychologists and psychiatrists with the necessary training and certifications from boards.

- **Advisories**: She had consultations with many specialists, realizing that selecting the best one would be crucial to receiving individualized care.

**Counselors and therapists**

- **Recommended Links**: In the same way that she looked for psychologists and psychiatrists, Sarah asked people in her network she could trust for recommendations.

- **Specialization**: She sought out experts who focused on ADHD or similar disorders to make sure they had a thorough awareness of the difficulties she had.

- **Therapeutic Approach:** After weighing the advantages and disadvantages of each possible therapist, Sarah selected the one whose techniques complemented her preferences and requirements.

## Communities and support groups on the internet

- **Local Support Groups**: Sarah looked through the yellow pages and contacted her physician to find out about local support groups for ADHD.

- **Online Groups:** She was an enthusiastic participant in online forums and groups for ADHD, asking other members who had good experiences with doctors for referrals.

Sarah's trip through the resources and support system changed her. She came to see that she was not alone in her struggle with ADHD; there were a plethora of people who could provide empathy and useful answers. Through the use of digital tools, online forums, therapy, and support groups, Sarah gained the ability to better manage her disease. She also received specialized tactics and knowledgeable insights from the advice of trained specialists, which enabled her to successfully negotiate the challenges of living with ADHD. Sarah's experience demonstrates the value of looking for and making use of the resources and assistance that are available to live a happy life even in the face of the difficulties that ADHD may provide.

# Chapter 10

# Advice from Young Adults with ADHD"

We have the honor of presenting priceless guidance from young people who have effectively managed the difficulties of living with ADHD in this chapter. These people have been there, done the struggles, and figured out what works. Their observations provide a plethora of knowledge to anybody on a similar path.

## Meet the Experts: ADHD Advocates

1. Alex: Mastering Hyperconcentration*

The 26-year-old designer and artist Alex discusses hyperfocus in his words:

"Your superpower might be hyperfocus. It's similar to focusing intensely on something you actually find interesting. Not everything is negative. Discover how to use it. Ride the surge of laser-like focus and productivity that comes with having a love for something. Just keep in mind to set alarms so you may take breaks and maintain your sense of reality."

## Olivia: The Influence of Acceptance of Oneself

Writer and public speaker Olivia, 24, places a strong emphasis on accepting oneself.

"The first step toward properly controlling your ADHD is accepting it. Consider it a new way of thinking rather than a "disorder." You have certain qualities that make you special. You may begin working with your brain rather than against it once you accept that.

## Michael: Time Management Techniques

The 28-year-old software engineer Michael talks about time management.

"Time management is crucial. Locate a system that suits your needs. Make a schedule using an electronic calendar or a traditional paper planner. Divide the work into smaller, more doable portions. Don't forget that using tools like reminder apps or asking for assistance is OK."

## Emma: Getting Around Drugs

Emma, a 22-year-old college student, discusses how to take medications.

"At first, I was apprehensive about taking medication, but it really helped me." Talk to your physician if you're thinking about it. Have patience; determining the appropriate drug and dose may need some trial and error. But if you do, it could alter the course of events."

## Liam: The Advantages of Habit

The 25-year-old businessman Liam highlights the importance of consistency.

Creating daily schedules for activities such as getting up, working out, eating, and going to bed may help to organize and lessen confusion. It eases my tension and keeps me organized."

## Grace: Support Networks' Function

Grace, a 27-year-old champion for mental health, emphasizes the need of having a support system:

"Never be afraid to ask for help from your friends and family. They could be the best pals you have. Tell them about your successes and challenges with ADHD. And get expert assistance if necessary. For me, therapy has changed everything."

## Daniel: Intense Mindfulness Practice

23-year-old musician and student Daniel talks about the advantages of mindfulness.

"Mindfulness techniques, such as meditation and deep breathing, may lessen anxiety, help you control your impulses, and enhance your general wellbeing. It resembles a mental fitness center. You become more aware of your thoughts and emotions with regular practice."

## 8. Maya: Getting Into Tech

Maya, a social media manager of 21 years old, talks about the function of technology:
Make the most of technology. Numerous tools and applications are available to assist with ADHD. They might be your hidden assets for maintaining attention and organization, from time management programs to reminder applications."

## Ethan: The Influence of Setting Priorities

The 29-year-old project manager Ethan stresses the need of setting priorities:

"You are unable to complete everything. Thus, set priorities. Decide which of your duties are the most essential, then start with them. The rest can wait. It's a game of prioritizing what really important at any given time and concentrating your efforts there."

## Ava: Dealing with Turndown

Actress Ava, 26, talks about overcoming rejection:

"You will experience rejection in life. That's all a part of the journey, whether it is professional or personal. Recognize that being rejected does not define who you are. It's a first step toward development and education. Accept it as a chance to become better."

## Mason: Continuing Your Work

The 24-year-old physical therapist Mason discusses the value of exercise.

Exercise on a regular basis improves mental health as well as physical health. It lessens impulsivity, increases attention, and releases endorphins. When you engage in a physical activity you like, it will become second nature to you."

## Mia: Creating a Helpful Space

22-year-old college student Mia talks on the value of a nurturing environment:

Tell your friends, colleagues, and/or roommates how they can help you. A setting that is supportive and understanding may have a profound impact."

## Noah: The Significance of Diet

The importance of diet is highlighted by 28-year-old nutritionist Noah:

"Be mindful of your food intake. Foods high in nutrients may significantly affect your mood and cognitive performance. Eat less processed meals, consume a lot of fruits and vegetables, and drink lots of water."

## Zoe: Sturdiness and Empathy

Zoe, a marketing manager of 25 years old, discusses perseverance:

Don't let failures depress you. Continue learning, experimenting, and adjusting. You'll figure out what works for you; it just may take some time."

## Leo: The Importance of Learning

29-year-old instructor Leo talks about the value of independent learning.

Recognize your ADHD from the inside out. You can handle it better if you have greater knowledge about it. Keep yourself educated, go to seminars, and read books. Your most powerful instrument is knowledge."

These young people provide a wealth of guidance for anybody facing the difficulties associated with ADHD, each with their own distinct experiences and viewpoints. Their knowledge emphasizes the value of accepting oneself, practicing self-control, and the strength of a strong support system. Through accepting their perspectives and incorporating them into your own life, you may forge a route towards accomplishment, personal growth, and empowerment. Recall that there is a thriving community of young people who have successfully navigated the road of ADHD, so you are not alone.

# Chapter 11

# Conclusion

We end off our exploration of the nuances of ADHD in teenagers and young adults in this last chapter. We've looked into the subtleties of this illness, covering a range of topics related to comprehending, dealing with, and living well with ADHD. Let's now consider the enlightening realizations we have obtained and look forward to the future with optimism and hope.

## Providing ADHD Empowerment to Teens and Young Adults

We started our investigation of ADHD by realizing that it's a distinct style of thinking rather than merely a diagnosis. It's crucial to keep in mind that having an ADHD diagnosis doesn't imply having restrictions; rather, it means appreciating your talents.

# Self-Acceptance: The Basis for Development

We discovered that the foundation of successful ADHD control is self-acceptance. You can work with your brain rather than against it if you accept your own thinking style, eccentricities, and abilities. Our young people have shown to us that having ADHD may lead to hyperfocus, creativity, and an alternative worldview.

## Successful Strategies

As we traveled, we accumulated a toolset of tactics:

- **Time management:** Developing a timetable and dividing work into digestible portions are just two examples of how this skill may greatly improve everyday living.

- **Organization and Routine:** Creating routines helps with organization and stress management by bringing structure and reducing chaos.

- **Drugs and Treatments:** Medication and treatments such as cognitive behavioral therapy (CBT) that provide people the necessary skills may be transformative for some people.

- **Information Technology:** Adopt technology to improve your everyday life and efficiency, such as time-tracking applications and reminder apps.

- Accompanying Networks: Rely on your network of friends, family, and/or professionals for assistance. It may be quite healing to talk about your ADHD and ask for assistance.
- Self-Care: Make mindfulness, exercise, and eating a balanced diet a priority.

They are vital to your overall well-being.

- Schooling: Find out all you can about ADHD. The best weapon you have for properly treating your disease is knowledge.

## Taking a Look Ahead

We must look ahead with hope and purpose as we get to the end of our trip. The options for teenagers and young adults with ADHD are endless in the future. As you start the next chapter of your life, remember these important lessons:

## Developing Adaptability

It's OK for there to be hiccups and diversions on the route of life. Taking on obstacles head-on, growing from your experiences, and pressing on are all parts of developing resilience. You possess the inner fortitude to triumph over obstacles and prosper.

## Aiming High

Your ADHD does not define you; you are able to follow your aspirations and make them come true. Your distinct viewpoint may be a valuable tool in helping you achieve your objectives, whether they are professional, academic, or personal.

## Accepting Development

Realize that development is an ongoing process. You're always changing, and the skills and understanding you've acquired from managing your ADHD will be helpful to you as you go through the ups and downs of life.

## Making Your Case on Your Own

It's critical that you use your voice. In the job, in relationships, or in educational settings, always speak out for what you need. Assist others in comprehending your advantages and disadvantages, and enable yourself to achieve success at your own pace.

## Helping Others

Your newfound understanding and expertise might serve as a lighthouse of encouragement for anyone who might be traveling a similar path. Be a friend, a mentor, and an advocate for those who need support and direction.

## Honoring Achievement

Honor your accomplishments, regardless of how little they may seem. Every success and obstacle you've surmounted is evidence of your tenacity and fortitude.

## Looking for Happiness

Finally, keep in mind that happiness is a necessary component of life. Cherish the times when you laugh, fall in love, and enjoy the little things in life that provide so much joy. Your experience with ADHD is shaped by more than just obstacles; it's also reflected in times of joy and contentment.

In conclusion, the path of adolescents and young adults with ADHD is a wonderful one, replete with successes, setbacks, and opportunities for personal development. As you go, remind yourself that you are not alone. There is a thriving network of people who are prepared to help you and who are aware of your journey. Using the techniques and knowledge you've gained, empower yourself and look forward to the future with optimism and hope. Your journey is unique, and there are many options. You have a special viewpoint that will help you achieve great things, and the world is waiting for you to shine.

Printed in Great Britain
by Amazon

40585002R00096